The CLEAR SKIN *Manifesto*

From Blemishes to Brilliance

By

KAREN C. SMITH

DISCLAIMER

This book is intended for informational purposes only. The author shares personal experiences and insights, and while every effort has been made to ensure the accuracy of the information, individual circumstances may vary. The book does not provide financial advice, and readers are encouraged to consult with relevant professionals for personalized guidance.

Please note that the content of this book should not be duplicated or reproduced without the explicit permission of the author. Any unauthorized duplication is a violation of copyright law.

TABLE OF CONTENT

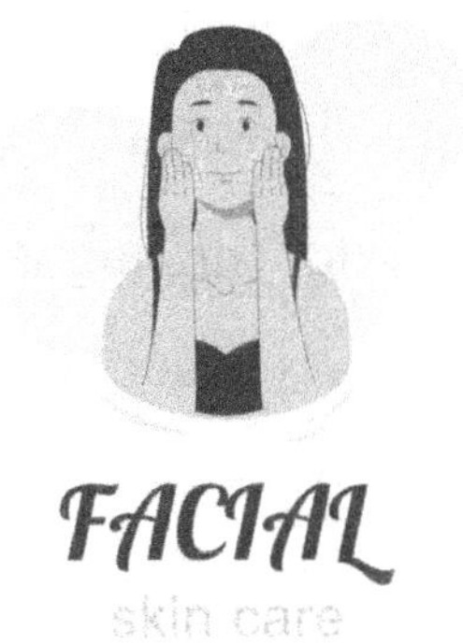

INTRODUCTION

Unveiling the Journey to Clear Skin

Setting off on the path to clear and bright skin is a transforming journey that goes beyond skin care and cosmetic routines. I welcome you to delve into the subtle parts of my personal experience in my quest for healthier and cleaner skin in this exploration.

This introspective journey through the complexities of skincare is not just about getting a perfect complexion, but also about understanding the underlying causes that contribute to skin health.

Every aspect of our skin's canvas, from lifestyle choices and nutritional habits to the effects of stress and environmental circumstances, is important.

This book aims to highlight the difficulties encountered, the lessons acquired, and the

progressive evolution of a customized skincare routine. The pursuit of clear skin necessitates not only external interventions but also reflection and self-care activities that promote overall well-being.

We will discuss the importance of consistency, patience, and informed decision-making in the pursuit of clear skin throughout this discussion. I hope to uncover the layers of skincare, demystifying the process and encouraging consumers to make informed decisions customized to their unique skin needs by drawing on personal experiences and realizations.

Join me on this journey as we unravel the complicated fabric of skincare, combining expert views with personal experiences.

CHAPTER 1

Understanding Your Skin

The Science Behind Blemishes

Skin blemishes, which include a variety of flaws such as acne, hyperpigmentation, and scarring, are mostly caused by intricate physiological processes and external causes. The interaction of sebaceous glands, hair follicles, and the immune system lies at the heart of blemish creation.

Sebaceous glands secrete sebum, an oily material that is essential for skin lubrication. Excessive sebum production, which is frequently prompted by hormone swings, can result in clogged pores. This, together with the presence of Propionibacterium acnes bacteria, creates an environment that promotes inflammation and the formation of acne lesions.

Inflammation causes melanocytes, the pigment responsible for skin color, to create more melanin. When melanin synthesis becomes uneven, it results in dark spots or patches on the skin, which is known as hyperpigmentation.

Furthermore, blemishes can develop as a result of wounds or injuries, when the skin's normal healing process may result in the production of scars. Fibroblasts, which are specialized skin cells, create collagen to repair injured tissue. The scar's appearance is influenced by the type and arrangement of collagen fibers.

Blemish susceptibility is also influenced by genetic factors. Some people are genetically inclined to increased sebum production or a stronger inflammatory response, which increases the probability of blemish development.

External factors such as UV exposure, pollution, and certain skincare products can aggravate pimples. UV rays increase melanin production and can exacerbate hyperpigmentation, whilst irritants can disturb the skin barrier, causing inflammation.

Understanding the science underlying pimples emphasizes the need for a comprehensive skincare regimen. Balanced sebum production, a strong skin barrier, and effective anti-inflammatory therapies can all help with blemish prevention and control. Ongoing research continues to unearth the complexities of skin biology, paving the path for novel treatments that target different components of blemish creation.

Skin Type Identification

Identifying one's skin type is an important first step in developing an effective skincare program. Skin types are divided into five categories: normal, oily, dry, combination, and sensitive. Identifying your skin type entails evaluating several factors, such as oil production, moisture levels, and sensitivity to irritation.

1. Normal Skin Type:

   - Features include balanced oil production, low sensitivity, and a typically even complexion.

   - Characteristics include few pores, a smooth texture, and a dazzling appearance.

2. Oily Skin: Excessive sebum production, which often results in a glossy complexion.

   - Characteristics: Enlarged pores, increased risk of acne and blackheads.

3. Skin Dryness:

   - Characteristics include insufficient sebum production, which results in a lack of natural oils.

   - Characteristics include flakiness, rough texture, and possible sensitivity.

4. Combination Skin: - A combination of oily and dry areas on the face.

- Characteristics: Oily T-zone (forehead, nose, and chin) with drier cheeks.

5. Sensitive Skin: - Characteristics include sensitivity to environmental variables, as well as a proclivity for redness and irritation.

- Characteristics: Sensitive to specific skincare products or environmental circumstances.

How to Identify your Skin type

1. Observe Your Skin Throughout the Day: Note fluctuations in oiliness, especially in the afternoon when natural oil production tends to peak.

2. Examine Pore Size: Larger pores may suggest oily skin and smaller pores indicate normal or dry skin.

3. Examine Sensitivity: Determine how your skin responds to new products or environmental conditions. Sensitivity might be indicated by redness, itching, or burning sensations.

4. Check Hydration: Dry skin might feel tight and flaky, especially after cleansing. Well-hydrated skin feels supple and comfy.

5. Take into account environmental factors: Climate, humidity levels, and exposure to harsh weather conditions can all have an impact on your skin type.

6. Seek Professional Help: Dermatologists and skin care specialists may provide a more accurate assessment of your skin type and recommend customized skincare routines.

Understanding your skin type allows you to choose solutions that address its individual needs, resulting in a healthier, more vibrant complexion. Regular review is recommended because factors such as age, climate, and lifestyle changes can all affect skin features over time.

Understanding and Addressing Common Skin Issues

The skin, the largest organ in the body, serves as a barrier of protection against the elements. Despite its toughness, skin issues that affect both health and appearance are frequently encountered. This investigation aims to unravel a few common skin problems, revealing their causes and potential treatments.

- Acne: Acne is a common skin condition brought on by excessive oil production and clogged hair follicles. Genetics, lifestyle choices, and hormonal swings all play a role. Treatment typically entails oral medications, lifestyle modifications, and topical treatments.

- Eczema: Spots on the skin that are red and itchy are caused by eczema, also known as atopic dermatitis. A weakened skin barrier, environmental factors, and genetics all play important roles. Moisturizers, corticosteroids, and avoiding triggers form the basis of management.

- Psoriasis is characterized by thick, red patches covered in silvery scales and is brought on by an overactive immune system. Skin treatments, phototherapy, and foundational drugs help in the administration of side effects and the avoidance of eruptions.

- Rosacea: Rosacea causes facial redness and noticeable veins. Stress, hot meals, and exposure to the sun are all triggers. Prescription medications, changes to one's lifestyle, and laser therapy can all help alleviate symptoms.

- Contact dermatitis is created when the skin responds to aggravations or allergens. Recognizing and keeping away from triggers, as well as utilizing effective steroids, are the essential treatments.

- Urticaria hives: Hives are raised, irritated welts that can be brought about by sensitivities, stress, or contaminations. Allergy meds, as well as recognizing and keeping away from triggers, are incessant strategies for alleviation.

- Fine Lines and Wrinkles: Wrinkles are brought about by maturing, sun openness, and way of life decisions. This can also be termed ageing skin. Wrinkles can be prevented through sun protection, skincare routines, and cosmetic procedures like Botox or dermal fillers.

- Dark Spot Hyperpigmentation: Hyperpigmentation is brought about by an abundance of melanin creation. Sunscreen, topical lightening treatments, and chemical peels are frequently used to get rid of dark spots.

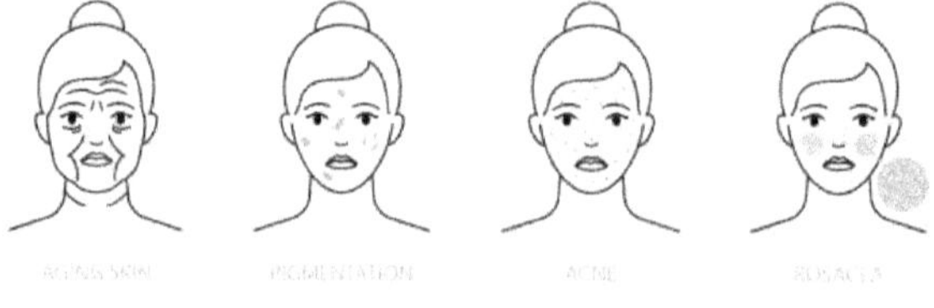

CHAPTER 2

The Clear Skin Lifestyle

The holistic practices and routines that support beautiful, healthy skin are at the heart of the clear skin lifestyle. For achieving and maintaining radiant skin, this strategy emphasizes a holistic approach to health, focusing on everything from balanced nutrition to adequate hydration to effective skincare regimens.

Taking Care of Your Skin From Within

Taking care of your skin from within is a crucial part of having a beautiful and healthy complexion. In addition to topical treatments, diet plays a significant role in skin health. An even eating routine high in nutrients, minerals, cell reinforcements, and imperative unsaturated fats gives the sustenance expected for solid skin.

Hydration is of the utmost importance. It's not just a cliche to drink a lot of water; It is required for healthy skin. Water helps get rid of toxins, which keeps your skin nourished and full. Consolidating food sources with high water content, like watermelon, cucumber, and celery, additionally assists with inward hydration.

Nutrients and cell reinforcements assume significant parts in skin sustenance. L-ascorbic acid, which is available in citrus products of the soil, animates collagen development, which further develops skin gracefulness and versatility. The skin is shielded from oxidative stress and premature aging by vitamin E, which is abundant in nuts and seeds. Vitamins and antioxidants necessary for healthy skin can be found in a wide range of vibrant fruits and vegetables.

Omega-3 and omega-6 fatty acids are essential for the skin's lipid barrier to remain intact. These supplements are bountiful in greasy fish like salmon, flaxseeds, and pecans. They reduce the likelihood of dry, lifeless skin by assisting in the prevention of moisture loss.

Protein, which is frequently associated with muscle growth, is also necessary for healthy skin. Collagen, a protein in the skin, can benefit from a diet high in protein. Lean meats, poultry, fish, and plant-based protein sources like lentils and tofu can help your skin's structure and collagen synthesis.

Finally, maintaining healthy skin necessitates avoiding processed foods and sweets. Consuming too much sugar can lead to glycation, a process that weakens collagen and makes you look older. Picking good feasts and restricting handled sugars assists with keeping a more adjusted and tough skin structure.

Habits of Hydration for Radiant Skin

Proper hydration is an essential part of a skincare routine for glowing skin. Water is essential for the overwhelming majority of body capabilities, including skin well-being and excellence. In addition to drinking enough water, developing hydration habits requires considering factors like water quality, lifestyle choices, and including foods that hydrate.

Since water is a universal solvent, getting rid of toxins from the body requires it. Hydration promotes the skin's natural detoxification processes and aids in waste elimination. Aim for at least eight glasses of water per day, adjusting according to the weather, your level of physical activity, and your requirements.

Take into consideration the quality of the water you drink. Reduce your consumption of pollutants and contaminants found in tap water by drinking clean, filtered water. Hydration is about more than just drinking enough water; the virtue of the water you drink can affect the general well-being and presence of your skin.

In addition to water, include foods that hydrate you in your diet. Oranges, watermelon, cucumber, and other water-rich fruits and vegetables help you stay hydrated. These food varieties supply water, yet they likewise incorporate significant nutrients and cell reinforcements that advance skin well-being.

Include herbal teas in your routine daily. Green tea, specifically, is high in cell reinforcements, which can assist with safeguarding the skin from extreme harm. Herbal teas are good for your health and help you drink more water every day.

Be aware of lifestyle factors that can affect how much water you drink. Things like drinking too much alcohol and taking in too much caffeine can make dehydration worse. Your skin will retain moisture if you reduce the amount of these chemicals in your routine and include more beverages that hydrate.

Take into consideration using a humidifier, especially in dry regions. Low humidity can lead to skin moisture loss, which can be aided by this. In the winter, when home heating systems can cause drier skin, adding moisture to the air can help prevent skin dehydration.

Finally, incorporate moisturizing products into a regular skincare routine. To secure in dampness and keep skin hydrated, search for lotions that contain parts like hyaluronic corrosive, glycerin, and ceramides. Reliable utilization of these things can assist you with accomplishing a smooth and brilliant coloring.

Stress, Sleep, and a Clear Complexion

Clear skin requires more than just skincare routines and topical treatments. It entails a holistic strategy that takes into account internal issues such as sleep quality, stress management, and overall well-being. Let's look at the interrelated web of sleep, stress, and clear skin to see how they all contribute to healthy, glowing skin.

1. The Importance of Sleep: Adequate sleep is essential for skin health. Various mechanisms critical for skin regeneration and healing occur during sleep. A sufficient amount of sleep permits the skin to create collagen, a protein that keeps skin elasticity and prevents premature aging. Sleep deprivation, on the other hand, can boost stress hormone levels, causing inflammation and worsening skin disorders like acne.

A good night's sleep also improves blood flow to the skin, supporting a healthy complexion. Sleep deprivation, on the other hand, can cause impaired circulation, resulting in a dull and fatigued appearance. Prioritize consistent and sufficient sleep each night to encourage healthy skin, aiming for 7-9 hours.

2. Skin Harmony and Stress: Stress is a silent destroyer of skin health. When the body is stressed, it produces cortisol, a hormone that stimulates oil production in the sebaceous glands of the skin. Excess oil, when mixed with dead skin cells, can clog pores and cause acne breakouts. Chronic stress can also impair skin barrier function, making it more vulnerable to irritants and infections.

Stress can be reduced by incorporating stress management practices into your routine, such as mindfulness, meditation, or exercise. These techniques aid in the regulation of cortisol levels, encouraging a harmonious balance that results in a clear and bright complexion.

3. Unmistakable Complexion Beyond sleep and stress management, food and lifestyle choices play an important role in achieving clear skin. A diet high in antioxidants, vitamins, and omega-3 fatty acids promotes skin health by lowering inflammation and increasing cell turnover. Stay hydrated to drain away toxins and keep your skin supple.

Regular physical activity not only relieves stress but also increases blood circulation, allowing critical nutrients to reach the skin. Furthermore, excellent cleanliness, the use of non-comedogenic skincare products, and the protection of your skin from harmful UV rays all contribute to a comprehensive clear skin lifestyle.

Finally, the pursuit of a clear complexion goes beyond external skincare practices. Prioritizing excellent sleep, successfully managing stress, and adopting a skin-friendly diet and lifestyle all contribute to a comprehensive approach to clear skin. When you embrace these interwoven factors, you will not only see benefits in your skin, but you will also enjoy improved general well-being.

CHAPTER 3

Skincare Essentials

Let's get started with skincare essentials! In this section, we'll go over the essentials for healthy, bright skin. Prepare to learn the keys to keeping your skin happy and glowing, from easy habits to the science behind it all.

Creating Your Perfect Skincare Routine

Creating your optimum skincare routine is a personalised journey suited to your skin's specific demands. Understanding your skin type, issues, and the important components that contribute to a thorough regimen is the foundation of an effective programme.

1. Identify Your Skin Type: The first step towards a healthy skincare programme is identifying your skin type. Understanding your skin's individual qualities,

whether oily, dry, mixed, or sensitive, allows you to select products that meet its demands.

2. Cleanse Wisely: Cleaning is an important part of any skincare programme. Choose a mild cleanser that eliminates pollutants without depleting your skin's natural oils. Cleaning twice a day, in the morning and evening, helps to keep the canvas clean for additional products.

A Simple Guide to Skin Cleansing

- Choose a cleanser that is appropriate for your skin type (e.g., foaming for oily skin, cream for dry skin).
- Splash some water on your face.
- Squeeze a little amount of cleanser onto your fingertips and gently massage it into your damp face in upward circular strokes.
- Pay close attention to any areas that have makeup, sunscreen, or excess oil.
- For eye makeup removal, use a specific eye makeup remover.

- Massage the cleanser into your skin for 30 seconds to a minute.

- Rinse completely with lukewarm water, making sure no residue remains.

- To avoid irritation, pat your face dry with a clean, soft towel.

- Keeping the skin mildly wet improves product absorption.

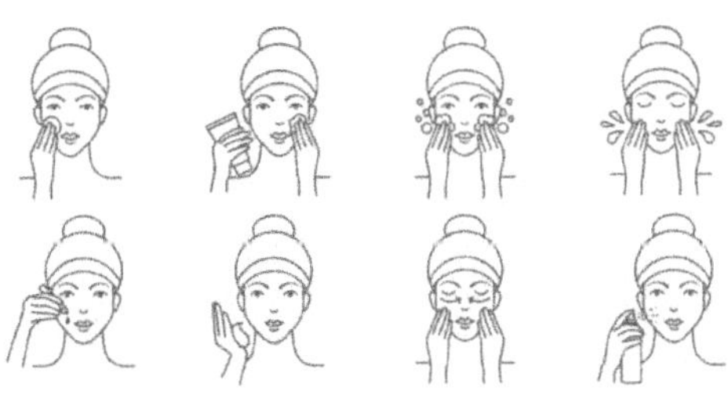

3. Hydrate with an Appropriate Moisturiser: No matter what your skin type is, moisturising is vital. Choose a moisturiser that is nourishing for dry skin, oil-free for oily skin, and lightweight for combination skin. Hydration on a regular basis helps to preserve skin suppleness and a healthy barrier function.

4. Address Specific Concerns: Incorporate targeted treatments into your routine if you have specific skin concerns such as acne, hyperpigmentation, or fine wrinkles. Ingredients including as retinoids, vitamin C, and hyaluronic acid can successfully address these issues.

5. Sunscreen is a must: Sun protection is an essential component of skincare. Even on cloudy days, use a broad-spectrum sunscreen with at least SPF 30. This protects your skin against UV rays, avoiding premature ageing and lowering your risk of skin cancer.

6. Gradually Introduce Actives: When adding new products or active components into your routine, do so gradually. This allows your skin to adjust and reduces the chance of irritation. Begin with a lower dose and gradually increase your usage as your skin develops tolerance.

7. Pay Attention to Your Skin: Pay attention to how your skin reacts to various products. Reevaluate

your regimen if you detect irritation, redness, or pain. Skincare is a dynamic process, and adjustments may be required to accommodate seasonal, stress, or hormonal shifts.

8. Consistency is Essential: Creating an optimum skincare routine takes time and effort. Maintain your routine and give items time to produce benefits. Patience is required for long-term skin health.

9. Seek Professional Guidance: If you're having trouble navigating the world of skincare, consult with a dermatologist or skincare professional. They can make personalised recommendations based on the needs of your skin.

Creating your ideal skincare routine needs careful consideration and research. Tailor your regimen to your skin's specific needs, be consistent, and embrace the path to healthier, more radiant skin.

Selecting the Best Products

Choosing the proper skincare products is an important part of developing an efficient and personalised routine. Understanding your skin's individual demands, finding crucial ingredients, and considering many criteria to make informed judgements are all part of the process. Here's a comprehensive guide to selecting the best products for your skin:

1. Recognise Specific Skin Concerns: Recognise specific skin concerns such as acne, ageing, hyperpigmentation, or sensitivity.

   - Look for products that have chemicals that are recognised to target and alleviate these issues.

2. Examine Ingredient Lists: Become acquainted with common skincare compounds such as retinoids, hyaluronic acid, vitamin C, and niacinamide.

   - To ensure efficacy, look for crucial chemicals and their concentrations on product labels.

3. Patch Test New Products: Before introducing a new product into your routine, perform a patch test.

   - Test a tiny amount on a hidden place for any bad reactions or allergies.

4. Consider Product Formulations: - Select formulations that are appropriate for your needs and lifestyle, such as creams, gels, serums, or lotions.

   - Take into account the product's texture and weight, especially if you have specific preferences or skin sensitivity.

5. Pay Attention to Active compounds: - Tailor your products to include active compounds that have been shown to treat your concerns.

   - Use retinoids for anti-aging, salicylic acid for acne-prone skin, and hyaluronic acid for hydration, for example.

6. Be Aware of perfumes and Irritants: - Avoid products with strong perfumes, since these might irritate sensitive skin.

- Look for common irritants that may trigger bad reactions, such as alcohol or certain preservatives.

7. Consider Your Standard Order:

- Recognise the proper application order for various products (cleanser, toner, treatment, moisturiser, sunscreen).

- For best absorption, layer items from thinnest to thickest in consistency.

8. Investigate Brand Reputation: - Look into the reputation of skincare brands in terms of quality and effectiveness.

- Reviews, suggestions, and dermatologist endorsements can all provide useful information.

9. Be Patient and Consistent: Allow products time to produce results. Skincare is frequently a progressive procedure.

   - Maintain consistency in your routine to assess the long-term influence of selected items.

10. Consult a Professional: If you are unsure or have recurrent skin problems, consult a dermatologist for personalised guidance. Professionals can offer items that are matched to your skin's needs.

Do-It-Yourself Skin Hydration Techniques

Keep your skin hydrated from the inside out by drinking plenty of water. Consider including hydrating foods in your diet, such as water-rich fruits and vegetables.

- Gentle Exfoliation: For a DIY scrub, use natural exfoliants such as sugar or coffee grounds. Once or twice a week, exfoliate to remove dead skin cells and produce a vibrant complexion.

- Make your own face masks with items like honey, yoghurt, or avocado. Masks should be tailored to your skin type, such as honey for moisture, yoghurt for calming, and avocado for nourishing.

- DIY Cleansing Oils: To make a DIY cleansing oil, use natural oils such as olive oil or coconut oil. Massage your face gently to remove makeup and pollutants.

- Tea Infusions for Skin: To relieve puffiness, use cooled green tea bags as an eye compress. Chamomile tea can be used to soothe sensitive skin and reduce redness.

- Natural Toners: As natural toners, use witch hazel or rose water. To balance the pH of the skin and tighten pores, apply with a cotton pad.

- Coconut Oil for Moisturising: As a natural moisturiser, apply a small amount of coconut oil. It is especially good for dry skin because it helps to retain moisture.

- DIY Lip Scrub: To make a lip scrub, combine honey and sugar. Gently exfoliate the lips to eliminate dead skin before applying a moisturising balm.

- Sunburn Relief with Aloe Vera: Keep an aloe vera plant at home for natural sunburn relief. Apply the gel straight to sun-exposed skin to soothe and moisturise it.

- DIY Stress-Relief Rituals: Use stress-relieving practices such as DIY aromatherapy using essential oils. Stress reduction improves overall skin health.

- Cold Compress for Puffy Eyes: To minimise under-eye puffiness, apply a cold compress made of cucumber slices or cooled spoons.

- DIY Hair and Scalp Treatments: For extra scalp health, apply a homemade hair mask made with substances such as olive oil or coconut oil.

- Sunscreen with Natural Ingredients: Make your own sunscreen by combining zinc oxide and a natural moisturiser. While it is not a substitute for commercial sunscreen, it can provide additional protection.

Remember that consistency is essential in any DIY skincare routine. Additionally, patch test new components to ensure they don't irritate your skin, and speak with a dermatologist before attempting DIY treatments if you have specific skin concerns or conditions.

CHAPTER 4

Nutrition for Clear Complexion

Foods That Boost Skin Health

A well-balanced and nutritious diet is essential for preserving healthy skin. Here are some foods that are especially good for your skin:

1. Fish with a lot of fat:

Fish high in omega-3 fatty acids, such as salmon, mackerel, and sardines, aid in skin suppleness and hydration. These fatty acids also reduce inflammation, which helps to prevent acne and redness.

2. Avocados:

Avocados are high in good fats, vitamins E and C, and antioxidants. These ingredients protect your skin from oxidative damage and provide a youthful appearance.

3. Seeds and nuts:

Almonds, walnuts, sunflower seeds, and flaxseeds are high in vitamins, minerals, and omega-3 fatty acids. They benefit skin health by supplying important nutrients as well as acting as anti-inflammatory agents.

4. Fruits and vegetables with vibrant colors:

Fruits and vegetables high in antioxidants, vitamins, and minerals include berries, carrots, sweet potatoes, and spinach. These substances protect the skin from free radical damage and promote collagen formation.

5. Tea, Green:

Green tea contains polyphenols, which are antioxidants and anti-inflammatory agents. Regular use can help protect your skin from the damaging effects of UV radiation while also improving overall skin health.

6. Tomatoes:

Tomatoes contain lycopene, a potent antioxidant that helps to preserve the skin. It also stimulates collagen formation and aids in the prevention of aging indications.

7. Chocolate, dark:

Dark chocolate, when consumed in moderation, can be helpful to your skin. It contains a high concentration of antioxidants, which help improve skin texture and protect against UV damage.

8. Yoghurt from Greece:

Greek yogurt, which is high in probiotics and protein, enhances gastrointestinal health, which is linked to skin health. A healthy gut can reduce inflammation and may aid in the treatment of skin disorders such as acne.

9. Extra Virgin Olive Oil:

Olive oil is high in monounsaturated fats and antioxidants. It moisturizes the skin from within, keeping it soft and lowering the danger of dryness.

10. Water:

While it is not a food, staying hydrated is essential for good skin health. Water aids in the removal of toxins from the body, keeping your skin clear and nourished.

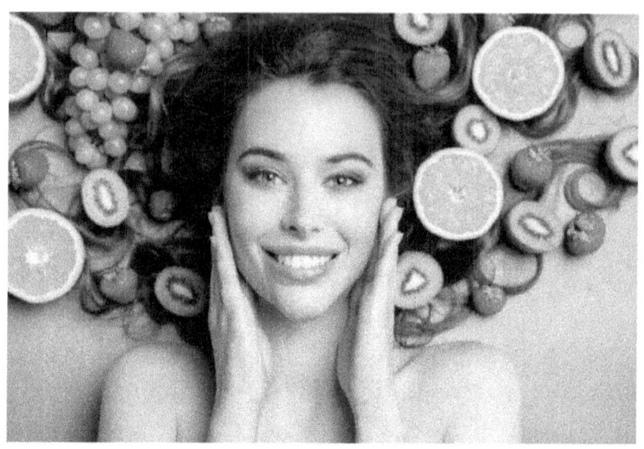

Incorporating these nutrients into your diet, as well as following good skincare habits and avoiding excessive sun exposure, will help you achieve a healthier and more beautiful complexion. Remember that individual reactions to dietary changes may vary, and it's critical to eat a well-balanced, diverse diet for good skin health.

Radiance Nutrients and Vitamins

The key to achieving radiant health and energy is a well-balanced intake of important nutrients and vitamins. These micronutrients are essential for a variety of physiological processes that contribute to the shine of your skin and overall well-being.

- C vitamin:

Let's start with the radiance-boosting powerhouse, Vitamin C. This antioxidant is well-known for its ability to counteract oxidative stress and enhance collagen formation. Collagen is essential for skin suppleness, preventing premature aging, and providing a young glow. Citrus fruits, strawberries, and bell peppers are high in Vitamin C, which can revitalize your skin from within.

- E vitamin:

Vitamin E, known for its intense antioxidant capabilities, is another mainstay in the radiant arsenal. Vitamin E protects the skin from environmental damage and aids in skin restoration. This vitamin is abundant in nuts, seeds, and spinach, and it helps to maintain a glowing complexion.

- A vitamin:

Vitamin A's importance in skin health cannot be emphasized. This vitamin promotes cell turnover, allowing new, bright skin cells to replace old ones. Carrots, sweet potatoes, and leafy greens are high in beta-carotene, a precursor to Vitamin A that promotes glowing skin.

- Fatty Acids Omega-3:

Include omega-3 fatty acids in your diet to improve your skin's radiance. These necessary fats keep the skin hydrated, minimize inflammation, and make the skin smoother. Fatty fish like salmon, chia seeds, and walnuts are high in omega-3 fatty acids, which help improve the natural radiance of your skin.

- Zinc:

Although it is frequently overlooked, zinc is essential for skin health. It aids in the healing process, the integrity of the skin, and the control of inflammation. Zinc-rich foods such as pumpkin seeds, lentils, and lean meats should be included in your diet for a vibrant and robust complexion.

- Vitamin B:

The B-vitamin complex, which includes Biotin (B7) and Niacin (B3), is necessary for healthy skin, hair, and nails. These vitamins aid in the overall health and repair of cells. Eggs, avocados, and legumes are high in B vitamins, which can boost your radiance from within.

In essence, a well-balanced diet rich in nutrient-dense foods is the key to releasing your inner radiance. While supplements might help, getting these nutrients from whole foods offers a more comprehensive approach to fueling your body and producing a radiant and healthy glow.

Meal Plans and Recipes for Clear Skin

A road to clear, beautiful skin entails not just skincare routines but also a careful selection of meals that nourish your skin from the inside out. Let's look at some clear skin recipes and meal plans that combine health with flavor to bring out your skin's natural radiance.

- Berry Bliss Smoothie Bowl for Breakfast

  Begin your day with an antioxidant boost. Blend mixed berries, spinach, almond milk, and a spoonful of chia seeds. Top with granola, sliced kiwi, and honey drizzle. This nutrient-dense bowl is loaded with vitamins and minerals that promote skin health.

- Avocado and Quinoa Salad for Lunch

  Toss cooked quinoa with diced avocado, cherry tomatoes, cucumber, and rocket. Make a lemon vinaigrette with olive oil, lemon juice, and a touch of salt. This salad is high in vitamins, healthy fats, and antioxidants, making it ideal for glowing skin.

- Snack: Parfait de Greek Yoghurt
Layer Greek yogurt with fresh berries, almonds, and a drizzle of pure maple syrup on top. Greek yogurt is not only high in protein, but it also contains probiotics, which promote intestinal health and improve skin clarity. This parfait is a delicious and healthy snack.

- Dinner: Baked Salmon with Sweet Potato Mash
A baked salmon fillet seasoned with herbs and lemon is high in omega-3 fatty acids. Serve it over sweet potato mash seasoned with cinnamon. The combo has a nutrient powerhouse, including Vitamin A, and C, and healthy fats, which contribute to a clear and bright skin.

- Snack for the Evening: Turmeric Golden Milk Latte

  Relax with a calming turmeric latte. Combine almond milk, turmeric, ginger, and honey. The anti-inflammatory effects of turmeric can aid your skin, and the warmth of the drink adds a soothing touch to your nightly routine.

- Hydration: Mint and Cucumber Infused Water

  A pleasant blend of water, mint, and cucumber will keep you hydrated. Proper hydration is vital for good skin, and the addition of mint and cucumber adds a delicate flavor that makes staying hydrated enjoyable.

Mediterranean Delight

- Greek Yoghurt Parfait for Breakfast

  Layer Greek yogurt, fresh berries, sliced almonds, and flaxseeds on top. This parfait contains probiotics as well as antioxidants and omega-3 fatty acids.

- Mediterranean Chickpea Salad for Lunch
Combine chickpeas, cherry tomatoes, cucumber, red onion, feta cheese, and olives in a mixing bowl. Dress with olive oil, lemon juice, and oregano to taste. This salad is high in fiber, vitamins, and omega-3 fatty acids.

- Hummus and vegetable sticks as a snack
Dip cucumber and carrot sticks in hummus. Hummus, which is produced from chickpeas and tahini, is a nutritious and tasty food that promotes skin health.

- Dinner: Lemon Herb Grilled Chicken with Quinoa
Marinate chicken in a lemon, garlic, and herb combination before grilling to perfection. Serve

with quinoa and roasted vegetables on the side. This meal is high in protein, antioxidants, and other nutrients.

- Snack for the Evening: Mixed Berries Smoothie
For a refreshing and skin-loving smoothie, combine mixed berries, coconut water, and a handful of spinach.

Glow-Inducing Greens

- Spinach and Feta Omelette for Breakfast

Whisk the eggs, then fold in the spinach and feta cheese. Make a fluffy omelette. Spinach is high in iron and vitamins, which help to maintain a healthy complexion.

- Kale and Quinoa Bowl for Lunch

Mix kale with olive oil, cooked quinoa, cherry tomatoes, avocado, and a lemon-tahini dressing.

This bowl is packed with nutrients and skin-loving elements.

- Almond butter and banana slices as a snack

For a quick and tasty snack, spread almond butter on banana slices. Almonds are high in Vitamin E, which promotes skin suppleness.

- Dinner: Asparagus-Baked Cod

Bake the fish with lemon, garlic, and herbs. Serve with roasted asparagus for an omega-3 fatty acid, vitamin, and mineral-rich dinner.

- Evening Snack: Lemon Green Tea

Drink some green tea with a piece of lemon. The antioxidants and hydration advantages of green tea lead to clear and bright skin.

Remember to tailor these meal plans to your specific nutritional needs and interests. Consistency and a diverse diet rich in nutrients are essential for obtaining and maintaining clear skin. Reduce your intake of processed foods, sugary snacks, and dairy, as they can all contribute to skin problems. Cheers to nourishing your skin from within!

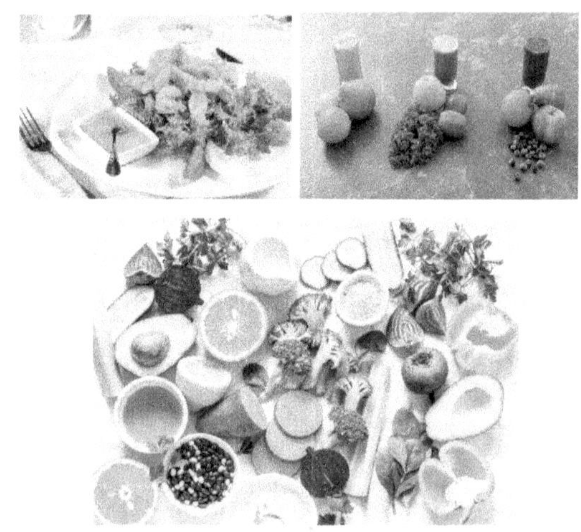

CHAPTER 5

Holistic Approaches to Clear Skin

Mind-Body Connection

The mind-body link is an important but often overlooked part of developing clear, bright skin. Stress, anxiety, and negative emotions can emerge physically, affecting our skin's health. A happy mental state and mindfulness, on the other hand, can contribute to a radiant complexion.

Stress Management

Chronic stress causes the release of hormones such as cortisol, which can increase oil production and inflammation, contributing to acne and other skin problems. Stress-relieving methods such as meditation, deep breathing exercises, or yoga help improve skin health by improving hormonal balance.

Conscious Eating:

Being conscious of what we eat has been shown to improve skin clarity. Emotional eating and the use of processed, sugary meals can aggravate skin problems. A balanced and nutrient-rich diet, combined with mindful eating practices, promotes general well-being and can help to cleanse the complexion.

Quality Sleep:

he mind-body connection extends to our sleep quality. Sleep deprivation or irregular sleep patterns can upset the hormonal balance and damage the skin's capacity to repair. Prioritizing consistent and quality sleep promotes skin restoration, resulting in a more youthful and revitalized appearance.

Positive Attitude:

Developing a positive attitude and regulating negative emotions can have a significant impact on skin health. Chronic negativity or worry can aggravate illnesses such as eczema or psoriasis. Engaging in enjoyable hobbies, practicing gratitude, and maintaining a pleasant attitude can all help to promote clear and vibrant skin.

Holistic Skincare routines:

Make attentive skincare routines a part of your routine. Spend time connecting with your skin, using products that elicit pleasurable feelings, and remaining present during your skincare routine. This thoughtful approach improves the efficacy of skin care products and fosters a sense of well-being, which is reflected in your skin.

Exercising for Beautiful Skin

Cardiovascular activities: Cardiovascular activities are essential for promoting bright skin. Running or jogging, for example, boosts blood circulation and hence delivers more oxygen to skin cells. This increased blood flow promotes a nourished complexion and can leave your skin appearing revitalized. Cycling is another fantastic cardiovascular activity that not only increases overall blood flow but also aids in detoxification through sweating, assisting in the removal of pollutants from your skin.

Strength Training activities: Including strength training activities in your program has numerous skin health benefits. Weightlifting, for example, boosts collagen formation, which is essential for preserving skin suppleness. This might give you a firmer, more youthful appearance. Bodyweight exercises, such as push-ups and squats, not only improve circulation but also help to get toned and healthy-looking skin.

Flexibility and Mind-Body Exercises: Yoga and Pilates, for example, provide holistic advantages for both the body and the skin. Yoga successfully reduces stress levels by combining movement, controlled breathing, and relaxation techniques. Pilates emphasizes core strength while improving general muscular tone and posture. These mind-body exercises not only help you relax but also help you have a more balanced and beautiful complexion.

High-Intensity Interval Training (HIIT): For those looking for a quick workout, High-Intensity Interval Training (HIIT) is a great option. Short bursts of intensive exercise not only induce sweating but also boost metabolism, which contributes to overall skin health. Including HIIT workouts in your routine might offer a dynamic aspect to your skincare routine.

Facial Yoga is gaining popularity due to its potential benefits in increasing skin elasticity. Specific face muscle movements help to tone and firm the skin. While additional research is needed, some people believe that including face workouts in their daily regimen helps them to have a more luminous complexion.

Workouts focused on dance, such as Zumba or dance aerobics, are a fun and dynamic way to keep active. These activities enhance blood flow and assist in reducing stress in addition to providing cardiovascular benefits. Dance's joyful character can have a great impact on your entire well-being, which is frequently reflected in the health of your skin.

Breathing Techniques: Deep breathing exercises, which are frequently associated with mindfulness practices, can benefit your skin indirectly. These activities lead to a healthier overall complexion by encouraging relaxation and stress management. Incorporating mindful breathing exercises into your practice can be a simple yet powerful addition to your skincare routine.

Outdoor Recreation: Outdoor activities, such as hiking or nature hikes, provide a double advantage. Physical activity is linked with fresh air and sunlight exposure, both of which contribute to general well-being. When exercising outside, however, it is critical to use sunscreen to protect your skin from damaging UV radiation.

Holistic Practices and Natural Remedies

Natural therapies and holistic practices can be a gentle yet effective way to nourish your skin from within. Here's a thorough examination of such therapies and habits that benefit overall skin health:

1. Hydration: Staying hydrated is one of the simplest and most important natural therapies. Drinking plenty of water aids in the removal of pollutants keeps your skin hydrated, and promotes a healthy, glowing complexion.

2. Herbal Teas: Incorporate herbal teas into your routine, such as chamomile or green tea. These teas are high in antioxidants, which aid in reducing inflammation and promote smoother skin.

3. Nutrient-Rich Diet: Consuming fruits, vegetables, and complete foods gives important vitamins and minerals. Antioxidant-rich foods such as berries, spinach, and almonds promote skin health from within.

4. Coconut Oil: Coconut oil has antibacterial and moisturizing effects. Topically using it can help moisturize the skin and promote its natural barrier function. Consider using it to remove makeup gently or as a moisturizer.

5. Aloe vera is well-known for its calming effects. Applying pure aloe vera gel to inflamed skin can help to soothe it, reduce inflammation, and promote healing.

6. Turmeric: Turmeric has anti-inflammatory and antioxidant effects and can be ingested or administered topically. Consider adding turmeric to your diet or making a DIY face mask for a glowing complexion.

7. Essential oils: Lavender and tea tree oil, for example, offer antimicrobial and calming effects. To address specific skin conditions, dilute them with a carrier oil and use them lightly.

8. Dry Brushing: Dry brushing is a holistic practice in which the skin is gently brushed with a dry brush before showering. This procedure exfoliates dead skin cells, increases circulation, and may help to smooth the skin.

9. Sleep Hygiene: Adequate rest is necessary for skin restoration and regeneration. Establishing

appropriate sleep hygiene practices, such as sticking to a regular sleep schedule and creating a calm nighttime ritual, benefits general skin health.

10. Probiotics: A healthy gut promotes good skin. Probiotics, which can be found in yogurt or pills, help to maintain intestinal health, which may aid the complexion.

11. Green Juices & Smoothies:

Green juices and smoothies with components like kale, cucumber, and celery give a concentrated source of vitamins and minerals for glowing skin.

.

CHAPTER 6

Overcoming Common Challenges

Dealing with Acne

Acne can be difficult to control, but this common skin condition can be managed and overcome with a consistent and holistic approach. Here is a comprehensive guide:

1. Gentle cleaning: Start by washing your face twice a day with a gentle cleanser devoid of fragrance. The skin may become irritated and aggravate acne if you scrub too hard. Look for cleansers that contain salicylic acid or benzoyl peroxide for focused therapy.

2. Hydration: Always apply moisturizer to your skin. Moisturizing the skin with a non-comedogenic product helps to maintain the skin's natural barrier. Even acne-prone skin

requires water, and excessive drying may cause oil production to rise.

3. Products That Don't Make You Cry: Look for products that are "non-comedogenic" if you want to avoid clogging pores. This diminishes the chance of extra breakouts.

4. Peeling Consistently: To get rid of dead skin cells, incorporate moderate exfoliation into your routine. However, excessive exfoliation may irritate the skin. Take into consideration products that contain either beta or alpha hydroxy acids (BHAs).

5. Specific Treatments: Utilize spot treatments containing chemicals like salicylic acid or benzoyl peroxide to treat specific blemishes. Apply these treatments directly to the affected areas.

6. Eat plenty of fruits, vegetables, whole grains, and lean proteins in a well-balanced diet. Consuming processed and sugary foods should be avoided because they may exacerbate acne and inflammation.

7. Remain saturated: Drinking a lot of water helps flush out toxins and keeps the skin hydrated. Hydration can help you have a more radiant complexion and promote overall skin health.

8. Stress Reduction: Engage in activities like yoga, deep breathing, or meditation to alleviate stress. Ongoing pressure can cause hormonal changes that bother skin inflammation.

9. Regular sport: Regular exercise can help you feel less stressed and improve blood circulation. To keep away from sweat-instigated breakouts, make sure to purify your skin after working out.

10. Abstain from Picking and Contacting: This is one the major issue since most people are tempted to touch their acne. So please and please, avoid touching or picking at your acne. Inflammation, scarring, and bacterial spread may increase as a result.

11. Sun Screening: Every day, use sunscreen with an SPF of at least 30. Sunscreen is essential because some acne treatments can make you more sensitive to sunlight.

12. Seek Expert Assistance: On the off chance that over-the-counter items are inadequate, visit a dermatologist. They can provide individualized advice and prescribe medications for hormonal acne, such as oral contraceptives, topical retinoids, or antibiotics.

13. Consistency and patience: Consistency and patience are necessary for acne management. Be patient and consistent with your skincare routine. Although changes may not be immediately apparent, persistent effort can yield beneficial outcomes over time.

Acne Types

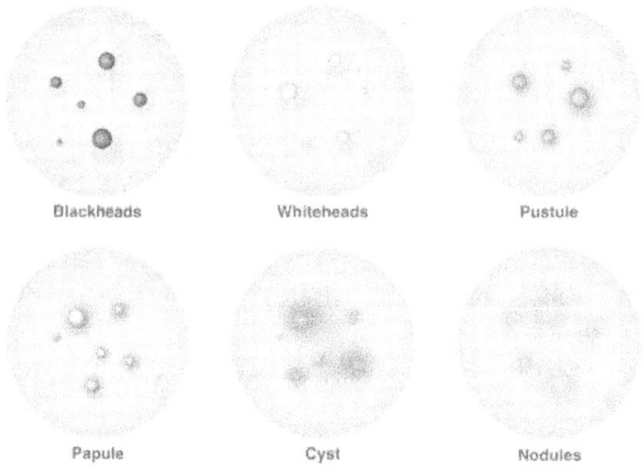

1. Whiteheads: Closed comedones caused by plugged hair follicles with oil and dead skin cells.

2. Blackheads: Open comedones are caused by the same circumstances as whiteheads, but the pore is open, exposing the debris to air, and giving the appearance of a dark spot.

3. Papules: Small, red pimples that do not contain pus. They arise when the walls around the pores rupture as a result of inflammation.

4. Pustules: White-centered pimples are formed by a combination of pus, dead skin cells, and germs.

5. Nodules: These are large, painful bumps beneath the skin caused by the accumulation of numerous, irritated, and clogged pores.

6. Cysts: These are deep, pus-filled tumors that might scar. They are the most serious type of acne.

Acne Causes:

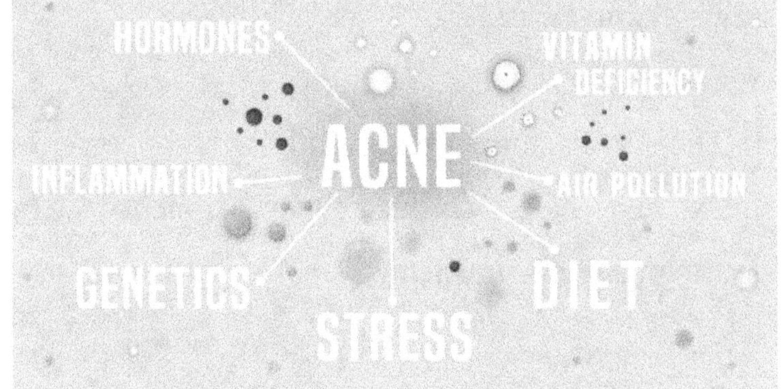

1. Excess Sebum Production: The sebaceous glands' overproduction of oil can block pores and contribute to acne.

2. Hormonal Changes: Hormonal fluctuations, particularly during puberty, menstruation, and pregnancy, can cause acne.

3. Genetics: Acne in the family can raise the likelihood of having it.

4. Specific Medications: Some medications, such as corticosteroids and lithium-containing medications, might aggravate acne.

5. Dietary Factors: Foods with a high glycemic index and dairy products may influence acne development in some people.

6. Tension: Stress, while not a direct cause, can aggravate existing acne owing to hormonal changes.

7. Vitamin Deficiency:
A lack of vitamins, particularly vitamins A and D, can influence skin health and contribute to acne. Vitamin A is important for skin cell turnover and preventing clogged pores, whilst vitamin D is important for overall skin function. A shortage of these vitamins may interfere with the usual

processes that keep skin healthy, perhaps aggravating acne.

8. Inflammation:

Inflammation plays a crucial role in the development and progression of acne. When the skin gets irritated, the production of sebum (skin oil) increases, as does the multiplication of acne-causing bacteria. Chronic inflammation can help acne lesions remain and raise the risk of scarring.

9. Pollution:

Particulate particles, ozone, and chemicals in the environment can all contribute to skin problems, including acne. Pollution, by depositing small particles on the skin, can clog pores, causing increased inflammation and oxidative stress. Furthermore, pollutants may combine with other elements like sebum and perspiration, resulting in an environment favorable to bacterial development.

Regular washing and pollution prevention, including the use of antioxidants, can help manage acne that has been worsened by pollution.

Managing Sensitivity and Redness

Overseeing skin responsiveness and redness requires a moderate and designated approach. A comprehensive strategy for reducing and preventing sensitivity is as follows:

1. Make use of mild cleaners: Use gentle, fragrance-free cleansers on sensitive skin. Avoid harsh products like alcohol and sulfates, which can dry out the skin.

2. Saturate consistently: To keep your skin nourished, use a moisturizer that is both hypoallergenic and non-comedogenic. Compounds like hyaluronic acid and ceramides can help maintain the skin barrier.

3. Test New Products on a Patch: Perform a patch test to ensure that any new makeup or skincare products you use will not irritate or cause

redness. Introduce one product at a time to identify potential allergies.

4. Avoid harsh exfoliants and abrasive scrubs: Avoid harsh exfoliants and scrubs that are abrasive. Instead, to increase cell turnover without irritating, use mild exfoliants like lactic acid or enzymes.

5. Sun Screening: To shield your skin from the sun, use a broad-spectrum sunscreen with an SPF of 30 or higher. UV rays can make people with sensitive skin more irritated and red.

6. Compresses that cool: Place a cool compress on the red or uncomfortable areas. This may help soothe and alleviate skin inflammation.

7. Utilize calming elements: Look for skin care products that contain soothing ingredients like calendula, chamomile, or aloe vera. These have anti-inflammatory properties and can aid in the reduction of redness.

8. Limit exposure to hot water: Hot water can dry out your skin and aggravate sensitivity, so don't use it to wash your face or take a shower. Use lukewarm water instead.

9. Hydrating Covers: Use hydrating covers with substances like hyaluronic corrosive or cucumber to give your skin an unwinding and saturating help.

10. Consider a hypoallergenic diet: For some people, certain foods can make their skin sensitive. Get personalized guidance from a healthcare professional and think about keeping a food diary to identify potential triggers.

11. Products Free of Fragrance: Pick "scent-free" skincare and individual consideration items to decrease the gamble of uneasiness from added smells.

12. Stress Reduction: Make use of techniques that reduce stress, like deep breathing exercises or

meditation. Stress can make the skin more sensitive and red.

13. Proficient Counsel: If sensitivity persists or gets worse, see a dermatologist. They can provide insight into potential underlying issues and recommend specific skincare products or treatments tailored to your skin's requirements.

14. Tests for Allergies: Think about getting tested for allergies if you think that some things are making your skin sensitive. Recognizing and staying away from sensitivities can further develop skin wellbeing decisively.

CHAPTER 7

Your Clear Skin Journey

Setting Realistic goals

Laying out reasonable and significant objectives is fundamental while setting out on an unmistakable skin venture. Here is a finished manual to help you effectively travel this way:

1. Self-Evaluation: Identifying specific skin issues like acne, dryness, or uneven texture is the first step. Learn about your skin type and what it needs.

2. Prioritize the Issues: Decide the significance and earnestness of your skincare objectives. You will be able to put the most pressing issues first because of this.

3. Break down the bigger goals into smaller ones: Separate major objectives like "clear skin" into more

modest advances. For instance, if acne is a problem, break it down into managing the ones that are already there, avoiding future breakouts, and fixing the ones that are already there.

4. Make a Skincare Schedule: Set up a regular skincare routine that addresses the issues and skin type you have. This might involve washing, conditioning, saturating, and the utilization of designated treatments.

5. Establish Deadlines: When estimating how long it will take to see results, be realistic. Perceive that getting clear skin requires some investment, and putting forth momentary objectives can assist you with keeping focused.

6. Minor victories should be honored and celebrated: Perceive and commend each achievement, regardless of how minor. You may find that sticking

to your skincare routine is easier with this encouraging feedback.

7. Change Objectives as Needed: Regularly reevaluate your objectives and adjust based on how your skin responds. Being able to change your mind about what works best for your skin is essential.

8. An All-Natural Approach: More than just using skincare products, clear skin is possible. Include a holistic approach that incorporates a healthy diet, plenty of water, regular exercise, and adequate sleep. The overall health of the skin is significantly impacted by these elements.

9. Consult a professional: Professional guidance is essential. In light of your skin type, concerns, and clinical history, a dermatologist can make customized proposals.

10. Keep up with Consistency: Maintain regularity in your routine. Skincare is a long-term investment, and the results frequently show up gradually.

11. Maintain a skincare diary: Keep track of your skincare routine, the products you use, and any changes to your skin in a skincare notebook. This could help you recognize examples and make informed decisions.

12. Give it time: Having clear skin doesn't show up for the time being. You need to be patient. Your skin may become irritated if you experiment with too many products at once.

13. Learn for yourself: Know what your skincare products contain. Information empowers you to settle on informed choices and select things that are by your targets.

Checking Progress

Keeping tabs on the development of your reasonable skin venture is basic to arriving at your skincare targets. To help you keep track of and celebrate your progress, here is a checklist:

1. Images of before and after: Take pictures of your skin that are clear and well-lit before you start your adventure. Regularly take follow-up pictures to see how things have changed over time. This visual evidence can inspire you and help you notice even the smallest changes.

2. Skincare notepad: Keep a skincare journal to record your everyday routine, including the items you use, any changes, and the responses of your skin. Keep track of your reactions to any new products that are introduced, as well as how your skin feels. This can help you find patterns and figure out what looks best on your skin.

3. Verify Your Persistence: Take note of how diligently you have adhered to your skincare routine. Understanding how your skincare regimen affects your skin will be made easier if you keep track of how well you stick to it.

4. Skin Journal: To keep track of external factors that could affect your skin, like your diet, stress levels, sleeping patterns, and changes in hormones, keep a diary. Knowing these effects can help you learn more about how your skin behaves.

5. Examine for Alterations: Regularly check your skin for changes in texture, tone, and the presence of particular problems. Take note of any improvement in skin hydration, reduction in acne, or evenness.

6. Item Adequacy: Analyze how well your skincare products work. Before evaluating the impact of a new product, allow it time to function. Think about

changing your daily practice if an item neglects to give the guaranteed results or makes terrible reactions.

9. Tolerance and Sensible Assumptions: Recognize that it takes time to clear skin. Be patient and realistic in your expectations. Even if your progress is sluggish, it shows that your efforts are paying off.

10. Appreciate and acknowledge Your Achievements: Be grateful for the things you've accomplished along the way. Your motivation will increase if you recognize and reward your improvement, whether it's fewer breakouts, improved skin texture, or more moisture.

CONCLUSION

"The Clear Skin Manifesto" is a comprehensive manual for accomplishing splendid and clean skin. Readers are provided with the knowledge and skills necessary to achieve their skincare goals by setting reasonable goals, adhering to a consistent skincare routine, and meticulously documenting progress.

Recall that reasonable skin is an excursion, not an objective, as you leave on this changing experience. Praise each little accomplishment, be patient, and put forth practical objectives. You can achieve clear, healthy skin by learning about your skin's needs, adjusting your routine, and seeking professional assistance when necessary.

In the final pages of this manifesto, let these lines serve as a reminder that your skin is unique and deserving of care and attention. Accept the flawless, brilliant canvas that you can cultivate. May your skincare journey be fruitful, potent, and a reminder of how beautiful self-care can be. As a tribute to your manifesto for clear skin, here's to the radiant, self-assured you.

www.ingramcontent.com/pod-product-compliance
Lightning Source LLC
Chambersburg PA
CBHW060951260726
48661CB00005B/1841